A New Way of Living

14 Ways to Survive in these Times

Sally Huss

REVIEWS

Sometimes you don't have to get over things, you just have to get through them.

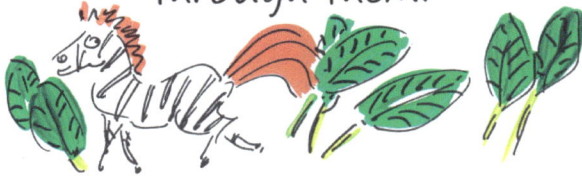

"Change was promised and change is certainly happening. This has left many people feeling very confused and depressed. Sally Huss's book offers an excellent guide to finding a positive path for the future. Sally's book shows us how to cooperate with these changes. Fighting to hang on to the old ways keeps us stuck. Sally points out that an optimistic attitude is very important. We may not be able to see the whole picture yet. She illuminates what is really important to us. She shows us how to look at our lives and discover blessings we may have overlooked. As we contemplate our blessings a sense of gratitude comes to us. This feeling of gratitude is an enormous magnet for positive change. We can transform ourselves and this is how the world will be transformed."

-- Carmen Scull

"Sally Huss has given us many books to guide children but this latest book is meant to inspire adults, be they parents or not. Our troubled times may make it difficult to see the good in everyday life but Huss has lots of practical suggestions. 'A New Way of Living' encapsulates Ms. Huss's very positive approach to all circumstances: life is a matter of attitude, pick a good one. No matter what crops up, it is important to remember that there are good things to be enjoyed every day – and good people to found everywhere."

-- Healthy Living

DEDICATION

For all those who strive to make a better world,

Thank You.

CONTENTS

Expect what you want, but leave the door open for something better to occur.

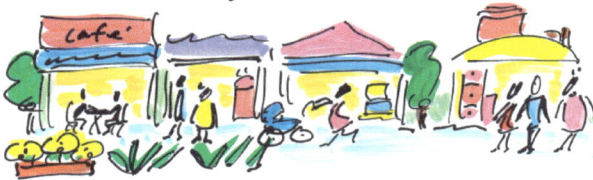

1 HOW IT APPEARS

There have been better times,
but none better to remind
us of what is important.

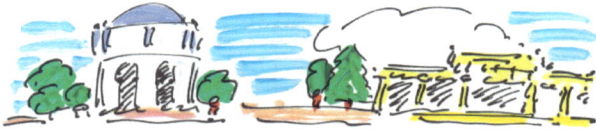

Now is a time of great troubles. The economy is in free-fall. People cannot afford to buy a home or afford to rent. Gas prices are high. Food prices are higher. Interest rates are moving up. The unions are fighting to maintain their power. Those with jobs are fighting to maintain them. The education system needs repair as does the tax system and the roads, bridges, and rail lines. The government is printing money with scant regard for the consequences. The security of the world is threatened by radicalism on all fronts. Countries are competing with each other. Those with money are buying up all the world's commodities without thinking of the vacuum such purchases leave for the local population.

Nuclear waste has become a nuclear hazard. Nuclear proliferation is increasing. Wars dot our world map. Gangs dot and damage our local neighborhoods. Illegals are flooding our cities. Women are abused and children are in danger of being trafficked. Extremism is in;

balance is out. God has been thrown out of most schools and civic centers due to the actions of many of our leaders. Churches and temples struggle to maintain a presence in society. Even Christmas has lost its tie to God. Drugs and alcohol seem to be an easy answer for those who want to avoid this reality, but they are not. What to do? How can we survive in this chaotic environment?

The first step is to remind ourselves that there are still magnificent trees to sit under, beaches to walk, flowers to enjoy, fresh fruit to eat, and good people to be found everywhere.

Yes, the world is in a mess but what is new? This has been said by every generation throughout history. This time, however, it is really a MESS! What should we do? How should we live? How should we raise our children? What should we think? How should we proceed? How should we begin again?

We must face reality. Life will never be as it was before. There will never be a chicken in every pot, the Partridge family living happily on Elm Street, or a car for every member of the family.

The American Dream is not over. It just needs to be revamped to adapt to the new reality.

Life is wonderful. Don't forget it! You might think otherwise if you look at the surface of things. However, this is just the surface. In spite of calamities and disasters, life keeps plugging along towards its ideal, its goal of balance, harmony and universal wellbeing. Change is inevitable. It must happen because the present state of mankind is intolerable. Life is unbalanced and deplorable in many parts of the world. So, change is good.

In today's world, nothing is guaranteed. Nothing is due. Entitlements are out, or on their way out. Responsibility is in. Taking one hundred percent responsibility for yourself and your life is the new mantra, the new way. Expect no handouts. Put your hand in your pocket. Put your thinking cap on and figure out how to survive! This means surviving physically, mentally, emotionally, spiritually, and financially. This guide is here to help you do just that on all levels.

This is a guide for a new way of living and a road map for creating a better world – for you and everyone else! Climb aboard. Start paddling. We are all in the same boat – life!

2 A NEW VIEW

*We suffer less by
understanding the lessons
we are undergoing.
School is always in session.*

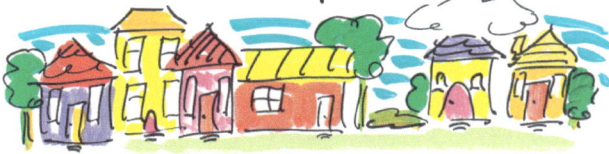

What we need is a new point of view. How can we look at these messy circumstances in a new light? How can we find a new approach that might give meaning to the chaos? We could look at our circumstances as if we were looking at a stage play – distant, removed, and unaffected. The players on stage act their parts from a previously written script. But who would write such a melodrama, such an X-Factor-sized thriller with high suspense, dishonesty, deception, and unresolved conflicts? The reality is that the players themselves have written each act, with the help of their lower natures. It is the actors themselves who have created this jumble of unpleasant situations. Either as countries or individuals, the actors have favored their own self-interests at the expense of others. They have created their own stories and plots throughout history.

Now how can you personally look at life from the point of view of your own wellbeing, without, of course, sacrificing the needs and opportunities of others? How can you make the most of what is around you? You have two available paths. One route is to identify with your circumstances and join in the misery. The other is to see your current situation as merely a moment in time in the long history of the evolution of humanity. It may not be the most glorious time, but it is a moment in time. By understanding that human beings are a work in progress, patience is required, not only for others, but also for yourself.

How then to make the most of it? That spirit within all existence and all beings, sometimes called "life," works toward betterment in every situation. It constantly seeks harmony, health, and growth, whether it is within a human body, an animal body, a plant, a tree, or an ecosystem. Now we have to see this striving for betterment in regards to society, specifically the human beings who make up society. We have to see this striving in longer periods of time. So, change will occur. Improvement will happen, even if it gets worse before it gets better. Life is forever moving people and things to a better place, towards its ideal – harmony. The secret to improving your own circumstances is to hitch your wagon to life – this ongoing, ever-improving force. How to do it? Love life in all its forms. Trust in its wisdom and know-how. But most especially, appreciate it for all it's worth!

So, here again, it comes down to a point of view. Be observant. Be self-protective. Be understanding that this is not the way it will always be. Love the life that you live and breathe now, knowing that the future will eventually be better. Until it does, you will be enjoying it as it is. In this way you will make better choices, attract better circumstances, and help write a more desirable script for the future – one with a kind and loving theme, one with harmony at its core.

Remember, there are family members to love, fresh air to breathe, cookies to bake, and good people everywhere.

3 A NEW WEALTH

Wealth is an unknown quantity. Anybody can be wealthy with the right point of view.

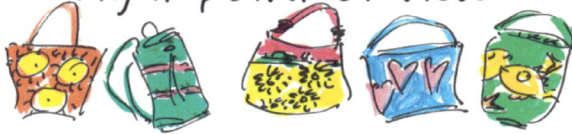

Wealth is usually associated with money. At this time money appears to be in short supply. The government, made up of our elected representatives, has been taking what it can from everyone here and generations to come, then giving it away in great gobs, trying to buy votes, friends, and influence countries. There is little you can do as an individual about this, except to vote for officials you think will do a better job. But personally, what can you do? You can take what you have or what comes into your family and value it. Money is stored energy. How can you best use this energy? First you need to separate the "needs" from the "wants" in your household.

This may be difficult when it comes to children. They are bombarded with advertising insisting that they need, and therefore must have, the newest game, see the latest movie, wear the hippest clothes, or eat the noisiest cereal. Kids play on the heartstrings, but now is a good time for them to face reality. Needs come first when it comes to spending. Their happiness must not be based on fulfilling their every desire. This is not possible now, nor should it be. Parents must appeal to the better nature of their children and include them in the process of using the family's resources wisely.

These times are tough and they require strong individuals. Strong, clear-thinking people are needed to set things right, whether it is in the country or your own household. Make kids aware of the value of becoming strong, responsible people. And, the way to become a strong responsible person is by making wise choices. Make a game of it with your kids, if you have them, or just with yourself. See how smart you can be with your spending. Try to delay buying something to see if that which appears as a need is really a need. Can you find it cheaper? Can you find it used?

Once you have separated the wants from the needs, you can focus on real wealth, and increase that. All those things that are timeless and do not disappear make up true wealth and can be expanded. The qualities of kindness, selflessness, compassion, generosity, truthfulness and joy warm the heart when they are expressed. A warm heart is a rich heart and one that enriches everyone. By encouraging your kids in these areas, you pass on true wealth to them.

Another area of wealth, which should be considered, is your personal wealth, the one you were born with – your health and all the parts of your miraculous body. Are they not priceless? Would you trade your eyes for a million dollars? How about your hearing? What price would you put on that? The sense of touch and smell are also beyond financial exchange. Your ability to move, think, and love are probably not for sale. You have untold riches within your own physical, mental, and emotional makeup. It would be helpful to point these treasures out to your kids as well, and teach them to treat these assets with due respect. Let them know how rich they are. These valuables cannot be replaced.

Wealthy is as wealthy feels. Add up your true wealth. Be sure to include your friends and family, your own physical make-up, along with your abilities, talents, and positive character traits. After that, how could you not feel rich?

Remember, there are mountains to climb, bikes to ride, songs to sing, and good people everywhere.

4 A NEW STRENGTH

Harmony never feels better
than when you establish it
within yourself.

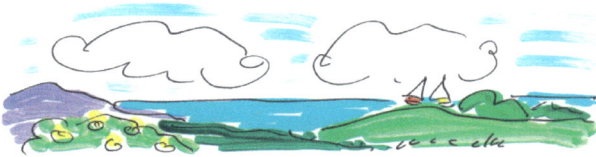

How do you gather the strength you need to handle the situations that confront you? Breathe!

Unknown to most people is the fact that the air we breathe is rich – rich in everything we really want or need to be able to do the things we must do. This includes courage, love, compassion, confidence, appreciation, forgiveness, gratefulness, steadiness, kindness, and even happiness. All we have to do is breathe it in. It seems an unlikely place to find help in difficult times, but it is there for the taking, and in great abundance.

The material things we need come to us by our efforts and our good fortune. Good fortune is that wonderful net of goodness that we have built within ourselves. It is made up of the beneficial qualities, virtues, and positive traits we possess. That goodness radiates outward and draws back to us a form of fortune. It may be a lucky meeting with someone who could lead us to a job or a better job. It might be a phone call that finally gets through to a potential client. It could even be a surprising lead to a new place of residence. These are our good fortunes and they are more useful now than ever. There is only one thing that can get in their way as they are flowing to us. FEAR! That is – psychological fear, fear in the form of doubt, lack of confidence, a sense of not being deserving, and other deflating attitudes or beliefs. These can shut down that net, take away the attraction, and leave us stranded. That is where breathing comes in. Simply breathe in what you need to dispel a fear, and good fortune is on the way.

Take a deep breath now and any time you feel ill at ease or stressed. The circumstances in our world today give each of us pause. Take the pause to breathe deeply. Our normal reaction to stress is to tighten up, pull in, and shorten our breathing. Remember the bigger picture, the one that promises change is in the works. This means that in the long run, even perhaps the very long run, it <u>will</u> be better. Your job is to establish a center of control, a solid base to work from emotionally.

True strength is found in this center and its essence is harmony. Harmony exists in a worry-free, zero-fear zone. Keep track of this network that is within you and make sure it is filled with goodness, so that the right kind of fortune can find you.

Remember, there are the songs of birds to appreciate, lawns to lie on, books to read, and good people everywhere.

5 A NEW OPPORTUNITY

Life goes on and on,
offering opportunities to
make it better and better.

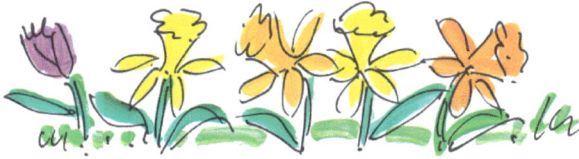

What are the new business opportunities at this time? Anything that helps people survive and anything that helps people conserve their resources or use what they have in a better way – are the new areas of opportunity. It may be in teaching or using techniques or skills you possess that make things less costly for others. It could be in exchanging those skills for products and services. The present generation of young people will have better answers to these questions than previous generations because they will have been born at a time of less material abundance. They will not expect to have everything handed to them, but will work to fill real needs for themselves and others. This particular time may be harder on those who are older, who feel they have lost something. The young will have lost nothing and therefore will be less encumbered   and   eager   to   improve   their circumstances. The ways and means they dream up will educate us all. Better ways to grow crops, better ways to purify our water and food, better ways to generate energy, better ways to maintain health, better ways to heal the sick, and better ways to educate everyone will be their areas of opportunity.

Just as the universe is moving us toward harmony, including realizing our oneness, our brotherliness, we appear to be more fractured. This is the life we seem to be living; however, we must keep in mind that we are moving toward a better life, a better way, a more fraternal existence. There are needs everywhere now. Where there is a need, there is a way. The young people will find them. Opportunities lie in fulfilling those needs.

Remember, there are lakes to swim in, rain to freshen the air, teachers to inspire us, and good people everywhere

6 A NEW THINKING

Look up. Brighter times are on the horizon.

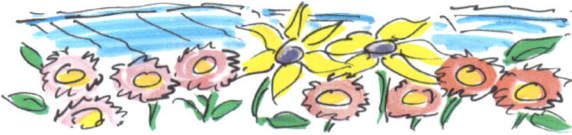

In the past it was assumed that if you went to school, got a good education, there was a job waiting for you. This was linear, rational, logical thinking. That was the way it was. But it is different now. Creative thinking is in and must be encouraged and used. Unlimited, uninhibited, creative thinking is becoming a necessity. This new thinking will open the doors to all possibilities of how to live, how to find work, how to feed a family, how to care for yourself and others in your circle. Basically, using it is how you are going to survive in these times.

The trick is to make use of your better self. Your ordinary, everyday consciousness is rather limited in comparison with your higher nature, your inner God, that is often called your "Higher Self." It is that part of you that watches everything, sees the best path for you to take and tries very hard to guide you to it. Intuition is its means of communication. Hope is its promise. Satisfaction is its guarantee. Harmony is its goal and the means to it.

Everyone is seeking something these days. The

answers are oftentimes beyond the scope of our rational mind. That is where your Higher Self, that smart cookie within, can be of service. To be in touch with a source that has a broader view of things and is looking out for your best interests is indeed a great asset. Use it! That wise, and always caring-for-you part of you, is on high alert at all times, waiting for the opportunity to help. Pay attention! Your highest good is the intention of your Higher Self. Trust and act on the intuitive impulses you receive. You will be glad you did.

To help you make this new way of thinking effective, here is an exercise you might want to try. Practice makes perfect, or near perfect. Aligning yourself with your Higher Self is as perfect as it gets.

With paper and pen in hand, find a quiet place. Sit comfortably, relax, and clear your mind. Focus on your breath, the constant on-going incoming and out-flowing of life. Appreciate this natural phenomenon that operates without your doing anything about it consciously.

Next, think about your main need and write it down. It could be to secure a job. It could be a place to live. It could be to have funds to pay bills. It could be a person with whom you would partner in business or in life. It could be another car. Whatever it is, feel how it would be if you had it. Make it real to you. Feel it. Make it authentic in the sense that it feels comfortable to you, nothing far-fetched. If it is a job, what kind of a job, what kind of a company is it? If it is a place to live, is it an apartment, a condo, a cottage or a mansion? To some, an apartment is a mansion. You are asking for help to fill your need at this moment. The feeling of having that dream come true is the engine that makes it happen. Now all you have to do is follow your hunches! You have set your need as your goal, your intention, your dream in stone in your mind as well as on paper. For sure the path to it will open. That other part of you, your subconscious mind, the worker bee within, will go into action to make it happen. You might want to give thanks that you have already received it. There is nothing like pretending. A little heart-felt emotion to go with your desire convinces your subconscious to go to work. It knows how to get things done. Using everything at your disposal, all levels of your consciousness, is the new way of thinking, the creative way of thinking. There are endless opportunities to fulfill your needs. You just need to know how to access them. Now you know how.

Remember, there is the sun to light your day, kites to fly, letters to write, and good people everywhere.

7 A NEW CONSERVATION

The best things in life are free and they are becoming more popular than ever.

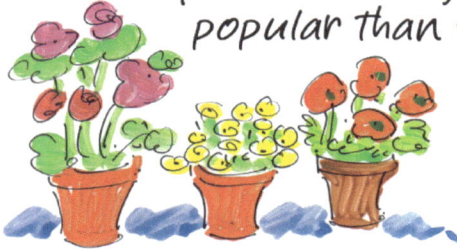

What do we need to conserve? Everything! In these times and the times to come, there is, and most likely will be, less "stuff" to go around and more of us to use the "stuff."

We live on a finite planet with limited resources. These resources provide our food, water, housing, and energy to warm our homes, and energy to allow us to travel, just to mention a few. There is not enough of some of these things to go around now and as the population continues to grow, there will be less.

"Greenness" is becoming part of our everyday language and everyday activities. Recycling trash, replacing plastics with more natural materials, driving hybrid cars, creating compost piles for our gardens, and other means of conservation are with us now. We are replanting forests, trying to clean our waterways, and are making an effort to stop polluting our oceans, as well as tamping down on manufacturing that pollutes our air.

As our population increases, and there does not seem to be a push to control it, waste management is becoming a challenge. What to do with all of this garbage – this throw-a-way, disposable stuff? We can start by using less of it.

On a personal level, how can each of us conserve without focusing on "lack?" It does not help to see our own resources as "half empty" or of not being enough to cover our basic needs. This point of view just sets up a "sorry" or "poor me" worrisome emotional state. There is a better way. The secret comes down to appreciation. Appreciation is love in its non-personal form. We must appreciate, that is love, what we have right now. We must appreciate it as if it were a gift, every bit of it.

Take money, as an example. In many cases these days, money is in short supply in households. How then to view the money you have right now correctly?

Money is stored energy. We use it as a means of exchange for goods and services. This stored energy can move products to you, such as food, clothing, cell phones, computers, gas for your car, heat for your home, water for your faucets, etc. It can also move people to help you, for instance, someone to cut your hair, repair your plumbing, hook up your TV, fix your computer, and so on.

We must now have a greater appreciation for this green energy (money) along with our natural "green" resources. Value it and use it sparingly. Use it for needs and for occasional wants, rather than the other way around.

If it is indeed stored energy, how can we conserve it? By using our own energy to do the things we would normally spend it on.

Can you grow a small garden where you live? Is there a community garden area that you could have a small patch of ground to work yourself? Do you have a patio or balcony where you can grow lettuce and other vegetables in pots or plastic containers? Do you have room for a chicken coop? Chickens produce the most perfect food – the egg!

Can you find someone in your family or amongst your friends who can cut hair? Who knows how to fix a computer in your circle? Is there anyone who knows about electrical appliances? These are just a couple of ideas. But again, the secret is not to enter this do-it-yourself mode with a poor-me attitude, but rather a proud-me one, by seeing how clever and inventive you can be, how capable and creative. Make it a fine time, not a fearful time. And when you do spend some of that great, green energy, do so gratefully, knowing that you are passing on more than just a dollar bill or two, but the effort from work you or someone has made. And in turn, you are benefiting the one who receives this "green energy" money for their use.

You might take up cooking, as a means of conserving your resources, if it is not your usual activity. Eating out can become habit-forming and expensive.

What did people do before everyone went to the movies or had a TV, or spent time on the Internet? They played games, knit sweaters, read books, developed hobbies, and they made things. They even spent time with friends around a backyard barbecue.

Where else are there areas of conservation within your home or apartment? Water? Water costs money. Air is free; water is not. Turn off the faucet when brushing your teeth. Take a shorter shower. Wash dishes by hand. Water is precious when there is none. Water is precious when there is. How precious is water? Our bodies consist of about 80% water. More than that, water is manna from heaven. It nourishes all living things. It washes and purifies us inside and out. It refreshes us on a hot day, and when heated, warms us on a cold one. Water in all its forms is necessary for us and all other living things. Now when you take a step to use less water, do not just think of it as a means of saving money. See it as an act of valuing one of our most precious resources. Be grateful when you turn on a faucet. Be humble in the presence of what comes out of it. It is no less than liquid gold! Without it, there is no life.

What else can you conserve? Electricity. Like many things that we pay little attention to, we do pay for electricity. It exists freely; however, it requires effort to harness and distribute it. That is what we pay for. Be conscious that you are spending money when you turn on a light or an electrical appliance. Is some of it wasted? Can you turn off unnecessary lights? Can you teach your children to do the same?

The role electricity plays in our lives is enormous. From lighting our world at night, to running our household gadgets, computers, TV sets, washing machines, dryers, vacuum cleaners, stoves, refrigerators, hair dryers, to our new electric cars.

In our towns and cities electrical signals run our traffic systems. Streets are lighted with electricity. Every business is dependent on the presence of electricity for phones to copy machines, computers, coffee makers, water coolers, etc. Be careful. Be grateful.

Where else can we conserve? How about gasoline? Probably everyone by now has figured out a multitude of ways to avoid the gas pump. Ride sharing, taking the bus, biking, walking, and staying home more are all ways to use less gas.

What we have taken for granted in the past must now be conserved and appreciated fully, just like the people in our lives.

Conserve friends and family. Care for each other and look out for each other. We are entering a time when we will become more and more aware of the brotherly nature of our existence. We belong to each other. We are one family and as such, we must conserve for ourselves, but also for others.

What else do we need to conserve? Conserve our own energy, our physical, mental, and emotional energy. Each day has a number of hours in it; use them wisely. There is little time for frivolous expenditures of time and energy, particularly in the use of your personal energy. Get rid of the things and situations that are no longer needed, as you move forward. Empty closets and cupboards of belongings that you no longer use. Someone else may be able to use them. You might let go of certain people in your life, those who drag you down or try to take you away from your goals. There is only room for positive, productive, constructive, useful people and activities. Then, be sure to give thanks for everything – every situation, every opportunity, every challenge, every bite of food, every glass of water, every breath of air, every friend, every acquaintance, and of course, every family member.

Remember, there are dogs to walk, birthdays to celebrate, gardens to grow, and good people everywhere.

8 A NEW EDUCATION

Struggles become us
when we face them
courageously.

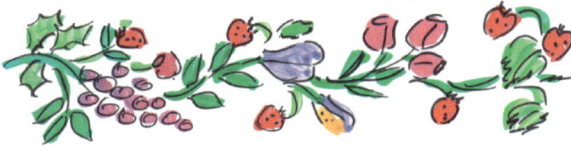

A new way of living requires new ways of doing things, and in turn, new ways of educating yourself and your children. Beyond the usual schooling that we all go through, we now need to educate ourselves in areas that may be unfamiliar to us. Acquiring skills of all kinds is the smart thing to do. From having the ability to garden, taking care of your own health, preparing meals efficiently, to cleaning a house or apartment thoroughly, to having the ability to handle electrical and simple plumbing issues, and all things computer related will be most helpful. These will not only be useful for your personal use, but as a means of barter.

The ways to market our talents, services, and products in the past was a well-established format. That has all changed with the Internet. Understanding the use of Twitter (X) and Facebook, and other social media platforms for business purposes has become a necessity these days. Just fixing a computer or cleaning it up inside has become an industry. Those who have these skills can always find work.

Besides using the Internet for marketing, it is a huge resource for information on every subject. Kahn Academy offers free tutorials on nearly every academic topic. There are practical YouTube videos on everything under the sun or about the sun. You can train yourself to paint, cut hair, prepare tiramisu, take pictures, give a massage, trim a tree, sew a shirt, write a book, create a film, clean a septic tank, etc. Practically everything you want to know is there, and most all of it is free.

The only skills not developed by the Internet are personal skills, those that are "in person" and not on line. Social media and electronic communities cannot replace face-to-face, person-to-person socializing. People need people. And children need children. Exchanging play days for small children with other parents gives everyone an opportunity to get things done, and allows children to develop friendships. Then too, make sure you are interacting with as many people as possible to maintain and develop your own inter-personal skills.

Expand education for your children beyond their classroom schooling. They need to be made aware of the importance of education in their lives. They need to be aware that work is a part of their lives and that there is a relationship between education and work. Starting at a young age, even as young as two, children should be given chores to do to make them feel a part of the "work force" in the family. They want to learn and they instinctively want to help. Give your children that opportunity. A few supportive words are in order for their efforts. "Good job, I'm proud of you" work wonders on a young person's developing self-esteem.

There are a million ways to add to your own education, by gathering skills, and developing your talents. The more tools in your toolbox, the more opportunities you will have to use them – some paid, and some for exchange. Learn as many marketable skills as you can.

The skills and abilities you develop can be useful for bartering. This is a time of not only change, but exchange. What can you exchange for what? What can you trade in skills or products for something you need? You may be richer than you think. Can you tutor a child of a neighbor for something that neighbor can do for you? Again on the Internet, there are sections devoted to bartering in your area. Your local paper usually offers a place for listing these opportunities. Let your neighbors know that you are available for various tasks.

Education is priceless. Keep adding to your repertoire. It makes you richer yourself and makes you better prepared to assist others. If we all learn whatever we can, there will always be someone in a group who can solve any problem.

Remember, there are changing seasons to appreciate, sounds of children to enjoy, lessons to learn, and good people everywhere.

9 A NEW WAY OF EATING

When one has little, one is grateful for anything. When one has a lot, one must be grateful for everything.

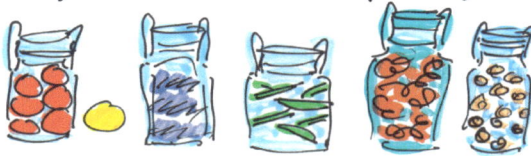

How can we change the way we eat that will help improve our circumstances? By making every bite count!

Food and eating have turned into an entertainment industry by our advertising giants. Clever people. Clever ads. But are they considering what is best for the consumer of the products and foods they promote?

We need to roll back the clock here and consider food for what it was originally intended – nourishment for our bodies. Our bodies cannot run on hype and hope. They need a variety of ingredients to help build and maintain our physical structures and keep them clean. This means pure, fresh, natural, pesticide-free produce and products, whole foods that have not been tampered with.

A wide range of pure, healthful, nourishing produce can be found at most farmers' markets. And, there is a farmers' market in nearly every town now. Even large grocery chains are providing sections for organic food.

Health food stores normally offer beans, grains, seeds and nuts in money-saving, bulk form. No matter what you and your family consume for food, the need to make the most of it is a part of a new way of eating.

You may not have thought of it, but there is another way to save on your food costs besides purchasing restaurant-sized amounts from Costco or making use of the multitude of coupons that are available. That is by making the most of what you eat. If you do, you will eat less. We humans have a strange idea about nourishing ourselves – that of getting food into our stomachs as fast as we can. No, real nourishment occurs in the mouth. The longer food is held in the mouth, the more nourishment is extracted from it. By chewing longer, the food particles are broken down, and the essence and vital energies housed in the food are released and made easier for the body to absorb. And in this way, less food is required.

Sending food too quickly to the stomach taxes the digestive system, which then has to break it down without the help of teeth. Then too, all the enjoyment of eating is in the mouth. Taste buds reside there. Textures can be discovered. The tongue can get into the act. Saliva helps release subtle flavors. And the nose can enjoy the aromas that linger longer.

It is better to spend time with one bite, than wolfing down a number of bites. Waists will remain trimmer. Appreciation too will increase if time is given to contemplating the origin of the food being consumed. Sun earth, and water all play a part in creating the fruits and vegetables that are grown. How far have these items traveled and how many hands have contributed to creating the meal that sits before you? This is something that should be considered. A meal is not just a plate of food. It is a whole wealth of colors, tastes, textures, fragrances, and vital energies that blend together to delight your palette and build your body. Even if it is a simple apple, it is a gift of life.

Every part of the human structure enjoys being nourished when dining, not just the physical body. A few thoughts about the contents of what is being eaten, engages the mind. Saying any form of "grace" warms the heart and sets the tone for overall enjoyment to take place. Life itself is a gift. Celebrate it at every meal by eating mindfully.

Remember, there are words to inspire us, friends to hug, trails to explore, and good people everywhere.

10 A NEW COMPASSION

The growing anxieties in the world must not touch the peacefulness in your heart.

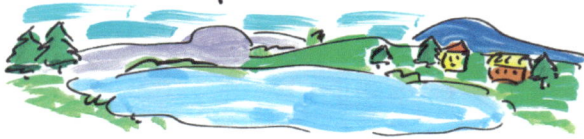

What we need at this time is a breath of fresh air, one that gives hope to all who need help. This is not a breath in the sense of oxygen. This is a need in the realm of spirit. There is much sadness that permeates the atmosphere now from those who feel lost, forgotten, abandoned, or who are jobless or homeless. Our shelters are full of people who need someone to care about them and give them hope. Our towns have lost their luster with stores, restaurants, and factories that have closed. We need a boost to lift the spirits of the people who live there, even if we are one of them. Now how to do it? Where to find it? The answer lies in the heart of all of us. The heart is that giving center that is always full of compassion. And it is breath that reaches in or up for what is needed. Reach, with a deep breath for love, strength, kindness or whatever is needed to help yourself or another. It is not a concrete solution to filling an empty restaurant for its owner, or of filling a store with buyers for a store manager, or finding a home for another. But it will help to lift the burden another feels in times of difficulty. It is a sharing of concern.

Give freely of your support in any way you can. Breathe in the compassion you need to give out the caring another needs. This is the new way – this is real comfort. It is the greatest of all help you can give or receive.

Do not forget that the air around you is filled with intelligence and kindness offering support for whatever you might need. It might be peace, strength, clarity, direction, or inner balance. The answers to your deeper needs and those of others are no further away than a breath of air. It is these deeper needs that really must be put right to put the outer physical circumstances in one's life right.

Remember, there are mountains to climb, poems to write, soup to make, hands to hold, and good people everywhere.

11 A NEW FORGIVENESS

Forgiveness is always appropriate.

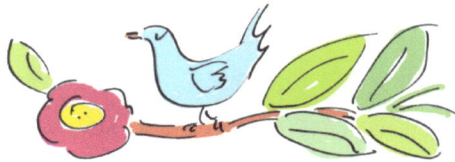

We are all looking for someone or some group to blame for the sorry state of affairs that we find ourselves in. Nobody is perfect or near perfect, that is for sure, unless your name is Mary Poppins (who proclaimed herself to be "almost perfectly perfect!") The truth is that we have maneuvered ourselves into this mess by ourselves. We are all responsible in some way. We have kicked the can of setting things right down the road until there is no more road.

When our governmental agencies do not act with intelligence and integrity, we can only blame ourselves for not electing individuals who will act in the best interests of all. When our corporations mislead those they sell products and services to, we still have the ability to buy or not buy what they offer. Yet amongst all this unprofessional and lack of brotherliness attitude, there are still high-minded public servants and corporations that act in the best interests of those they serve. However in many cases, there is not appropriate oversight to keep government agencies, institutions, and private corporations operating ethically. But why should there need to be oversight, if each of us has our own "inner sight?" We all know, deep down inside, the difference between right and wrong, and what the right thing to do is. It is a question of doing it

Instead, we have created a whole industry of educated men and women focused on "blame" rather than on "truth." The business of law has become just that – a business – not a venue for justice. Many of the structures around the world, both politically and economically, are collapsing because they are simply unjust. Again, whom do we blame?

Whom do we blame in our personal lives if our job is lost, or our home is being foreclosed on, or if the taxes in our state make it prohibitive to open a business? Who is responsible for our not being able to send our children to summer camp, or to school in presentable clothes, or just pay our everyday bills?

There is enough blame to go around, but it still gets you nowhere, even with an attorney. It is far better to spend your energy solving your existing problems than trying to find a scapegoat. But first, the blame, even if it is directed toward you, must be removed.

The way to do this is to forgive everyone, including yourself. This may not be easy, but it is necessary. One of the spiritual leaders in Hawaii (Howard Wills) has a poem that releases this energy. You might want to write it down And read it out loud several times a day until you feel that you hold no blame. Here it is:

I forgive you, all of you. Please forgive me, all of you. Let's all forgive ourselves, all of us.

Not everyone in a position of authority or decision-making, whether running a country or a household, sees clearly enough to do what is best at all times, even if their intent is to do what is good. So, you must look out for yourself and your family. Look ahead, stay flexible, see if trouble is coming, and where there are avenues to take in order to avoid pitfalls.

The errors that people make come from a lack of understanding of the big picture. We are at a time where human beings are evolving from a selfish animal state to a higher one. It is just a bit bumpy on the climb. Not everyone is on the same page, the one that includes peace, harmony, and prosperity for all. But you can be there. First, forgive and then give thanks. Give thanks that times are "a changin'". When blame is replaced by love, good things follow. Love the messy situations and difficult times because they will make you stronger, more alert and better able to deal with the future. It is because of the challenges, that you climb higher. Say "Thank You."

Remember, there are feet to tickle, dances to dance, games to play, sandwiches to make, and good people everywhere.

12 A NEW MORALITY

In these times, keep your standards high and your expenses low, and you'll continue to sail.

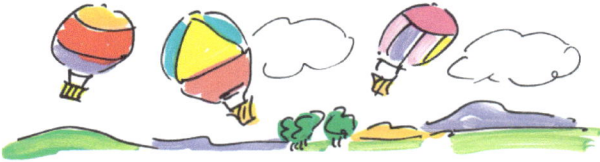

Our popular culture has taken us off track, and so we are living the script that has come from the morality of that culture. It is a morality based on winning at all cost, where extremism is worshipped, vulgarity is in, integrity has no foothold, and "me" comes before "you." It is a culture in which there is no shame in wrong-doing, violence is tolerated, consequences for bad behavior are almost non-existent, and growing potential disasters are being sweep under the rug.

Well, time is up. A new morality must evolve. It is one based on common sense and goodness. Man in all his many aspects has basically two natures – his higher nature and his lower nature. His lower nature has just about drowned out the higher one at present. But take heart, life is forever evolving and so is man. We, as human beings, are working our way upward. We are letting go of our selfish, animalistic ways and setting on a better path that will lead to a new morality.

Why wait? You and yours can live with integrity, kindness, a sense of justice, truthfulness, compassion, and love right now. In fact, it is essential that you do. Our new script depends upon it.

Long ago, people had little mottos to live by, whether they were raised within a Judeo-Christian tradition or not. The Boy Scouts, Girl Scouts, Cub Scouts and Brownies taught them. Alcoholics Anonymous taught them and still does. These were truisms based on spiritual laws. Those laws never cease to operate. The Golden Rule was the cornerstone for a child's actions – "Do unto others as you would have them do unto you." So simple, yet so meaningful. We do not need to go back in time, but go back to those universal principles and bring them forward. Be self-sufficient. Be responsible, and when your cup runneth over, share.

A truly moral person carries within his being great power, and commands respect. A truly moral person uplifts all others. We can all be such a person, in good times and bad, by not wavering in our commitment to high ideals. We all know what they are. They are inbred. They just need not be pushed aside by flashier, more popular concepts that grab our attention and build our egos.

Truthfulness, kindness, helpfulness, accountability, courage, compassion, forgiveness, gentleness, loyalty, patience, selflessness, strength, tolerance, and wisdom belong to that list of ideals. Teach them to your kids, if you have kids. Teach them when they are very young. Help them understand that there are consequences to their actions. Their moral structure will determine those actions, and therefore the consequences. We need to build a new morality. It will only be done one child at a time, one person at a time.

Here are a few mottos, or life thoughts that may be good reminders for you or your children as we all build this new morality. Copy them, then paste or stick them around your home or workspace. Make up your own. They reflect and encourage the development of these high ideals. It is where we are going, might as well get started!

*Kindness is good. Kindness is wise. Kindness is necessary.

*Focus on the positive and the rest will fall away from lack of interest.

*Attitude is everything. Pick a good one.

*Treated gently things become gentle, even people.

*Each day is a lifetime to be lived fully, joyfully, and without regret.

*Take each day as it comes. It comes perfectly.

*Be pleased with what life serves you and you will be pleasantly surprised by dessert.

*Your worth is invaluable. Your know it is priceless.

*How you consider the gift of life you have been given determines everything.

*Settle down with harmony and live happily ever after.

*A person who is like the sun, shining equally on everyone, is very great indeed.

*Dream big, work hard, smile always and good things will happen.

Remember, there are games to play, soup to sip, ducks to feed, and good people everywhere.

13 A NEW HAPPINESS

Happiness that depends on happenings is short-lived. Happiness that depends on nothing is forever.

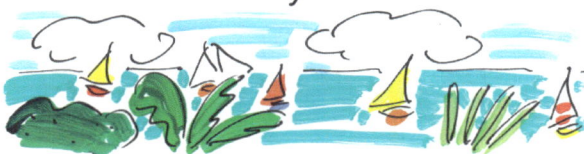

Our new happiness needs to be based on enjoying what we do and not on what we have or get. We should make every effort to enjoy ourselves regardless of circumstances. Circumstances will change continuously, some for the better, some for the worse. Training ourselves to enjoy it all is the new way to happiness.

To enrich our lives with our attitude, rather than with things is a handy trick, especially when there may be fewer things we are able to purchase. More often than not, we wait to get something or be with someone before we are happy. *However, if we wait to be happy, we will wait forever. If we can be happy now, we will be happy forever.* This is one of the most important things you can master yourself and teach your children – how to be happy now with what you have. This doesn't mean you do not encourage yourself or your kids to strive for more. It is just that happiness is not about getting more. By focusing on happiness in this way, you will be reminding yourself of something that you may have forgotten – that the state of happiness is your true nature.

And how do you do it? How do you become happy when circumstances become difficult? Easy – CHOOSE! *Happy days are made by happy people; happy people are made by choice.* Sometimes we forget that we have the ability to choose. It is one of the gifts given to us at birth. It is oftentimes suppressed by our upbringing and environment; however, it is always there. Use it!

Live happy, life is better that way.

Happiness, as you may have discovered, has a certain beauty to it. You can see it in others. You can develop it in yourself. Just as more opportunities come to those who are beautiful, more opportunities come to those who are beautifully happy.

You can be one of the "beautiful people" by developing this quality within yourself. Happiness is a skill, a habit that can be developed and mastered. It has unlimited positive consequences in your life and those around you – and, it's free! So don't hold back in the happiness area, give it your all. As you do, you will find that you feel infinitely better for having adopted this amazing point of view. The happiness you spread to others runs through you first. There is just no end to the benefits of a happy attitude. Jump in!

Remember, there are clouds to daydream on, sketches to make, apples to eat, butterflies to admire, and good people everywhere.

14 A NEW LIFE

*Beyond our knowing is
a caring so vast that
our small presence is still
considered important.*

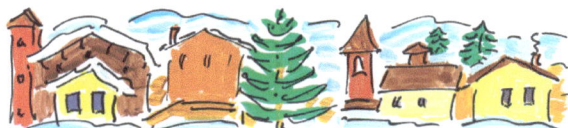

Finding a way into this new way of living takes some practice, some dedication, some creativity, and some adjustment. Change may not be easy, but it can be exciting. Make it an adventure. Develop new tools. Expand your view of how to live to one that includes adaptability and innovation. You can more than survive; you can thrive in these times and those ahead by being open and positive. Keep harmony as your keystone. Look forward, laugh a lot, and let life do the maneuvering. Place your needs ahead of your wants until your wants become your needs. Then, see how much life loves you by the gifts it sends your way, including the challenges that build your character and strength. You will be surprised at how wonderful life is and how great you can become. It may not be greatness in the world, but rather greatness in the world within.

If we can be examples to others during difficult times, they too will see the usefulness of being positive and happy. We are one family, the family of man. Take care of your personal family and yourself first by using these survival tools and others that you create. Then, reach out with your thoughts, wishes, and actions to assist your brothers and sisters. All manner of good things will return to you. Life is nothing more than a mirror, showing us ourselves by the circumstances that unfold around us. As you stand before it, be the qualities that you want to see in your future. It is a new stage, a new play, and you are one of the actors writing the script. Take what you have learned here in this survival guide and title this play "Life is Wonderful!" And so, it will be – a new way of living!

* * * **

ABOUT THE AUTHOR

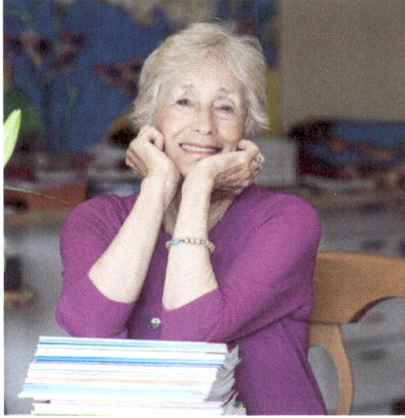

Sally Huss

"Bright and happy," "light and whimsical" have been the catch phrases attached to the writings and art of Sally Huss for over 40 years.

After graduating from USC with a degree in Fine Art, Sally married Marv Huss (formerly a top executive with Hallmark Cards). The two created 26 Sally Huss Galleries across the country filled with Sally's creations.

Presently, Sally writes and illustrates children's books (over 100), plus books on pickleball, tennis, and life. Her King Features syndicated panel, Happy Musings, offers delightful thoughts to brighten any day.

Formerly, Sally was a Wimbledon semi-finalist and National and Wimbledon Junior Champion.

www.sallyhuss.com

www.ingramcontent.com/pod-product-compliance
Lightning Source LLC
Chambersburg PA
CBHW041227270326
41934CB00004B/188